Plant Power Foods

100 Delicious Recipes

Plant Based Foods Can Work Wonders For Your Health

Barbara Williams

Disclaimer

Table of Contents

Introduction

Plant based foods are rich in antioxidants that prevent diseases and work wonders by boosting your immune system and ensuring that your body's metabolism works the way it should. It contains carotenoids, flavonoids and phytoestrogen among other vital properties that will work wonders for your health.

Plant Power Foods are packed with phytochemicals that are good sources of calcium, magnesium, potassium, fiber, iron phosphorus, folic acid, iron, zinc, selenium, essential amino acids, vitamins A, B, C and E, all of which are vital to our health. Many of the plant based foods included in these recipes are packed with antioxidants, beta carotene, chlorophyll, iron and essential fatty acids.

When you eat meat-based diets and processed foods, the body gets overworked trying to digest the foods and eliminate the toxins. As a result, the body speaks to you in form of illnesses and diseases caused by the toxins and the extra work the body needs in eliminating these foods. The body's metabolism slows down and loses the ability to fight illnesses.

There are many people who have allergies and food intolerances to meat-based foods but when they switch to plant based foods, these problems resolve themselves. Diet has a major part to play in arthritis, diabetes, cardiovascular diseases, obesity, cancer and other diseases. People who suffer from these conditions react well to plant power foods. This is because many diseases are caused by inflammation. Take for example arthritis. This is an auto-immune disease that affects the joints, bones and muscles.

When someone has arthritis, the joints become inflamed and there is pain, swelling and inflammation. Arthritis affects all age groups although it is progressive. The condition has no cure and it is usually managed. There are many different types of arthritis but the most common ones are rheumatoid arthritis and osteoarthritis.

Osteoarthritis affects mainly the cartridge lining of the joints especially the smooth part and it eats it away as it progresses. The disease usually affects the knees and hips but it can also affect other joints. Knee and hip replacement are common among people suffering from osteoarthritis to ease pain and disability. If you have arthritis, you may have flare-ups when you eat certain foods.

When you get a flare-up, stop eating the food for some days and try to eat the food and if you still get flare-ups then stop eating the food altogether. Milk, cheese, cream, wheat and wheat products, meat and eggs are some of the foods that cause inflammation in some people. Some people are allergic to dairy products like milk, while others are allergic to meat, wheat and other products.

Take plant power foods if you want to live a long and vibrant life. You can never go wrong with the Delicious Plant based Diets described in this book.

1: Why Plant Power Foods are the Best

- Plant power foods contain phytonutrients which the body uses to prevent and fight diseases.

- Carotenoids are found in red, yellow, purple pigmented fruits and vegetables and deep rich colored fruits and vegetables which include tomatoes, spinach, strawberries, raspberries, blueberries, cherries, plums, oranges, tangerines, watermelon, carrots, bell peppers, broccoli and others.

- Flavonoid-rich foods include apples, berries, onions, green teas among others.

- Pytoestrogens are found in growing plants like sprouts and in berries, flaxseed, linseed, pulses, beans, whole grains, fruits and vegetables.

You will get all the foods you require in plant based diets

Proteins

There are many sources of proteins in plant power foods unlike what many people think. These include beans, nuts, lentils, quinoa, seeds, soya foods, sprouts, chia, leafy green vegetables and spirulina. So there is no way your diet can lack proteins. Proteins build muscles and help to repair our bodies.

Carbohydrates

There are many sources of carbohydrates which include barley, brown rice, oats, potatoes, sweet potatoes, arrow-roots, yams, flaxseed, linseed, whole grains, whole-meal wheat and pastas. Carbohydrates are your energy-giving foods.

Vitamins and Minerals

Many fruits and vegetables and other plants are loaded with vitamins and minerals which the body needs to function properly. These are found in green leafy vegetables like spinach and collard greens, cruciferous vegetables like cabbage and broccoli, carrots, bell peppers, onions, celery, asparagus, tomatoes and fruits such as berries, apples, apricots, pears kiwi, melon, watermelon, bananas, papaya and mangos among many others.

Vitamin C fights against infections, B Vitamins help to synthesize white blood cells which are your defense against illnesses and diseases. Vitamin K found in vegetables like kale help in the clotting of the blood.

You need calcium and Vitamin D to make your bones and teeth strong and avoid the risks associated with osteoporosis. Vitamin D helps in the absorption of calcium. Leafy green vegetables like spinach and collard greens contain calcium. You can add them to your smoothies or cook them lightly. Spinach is rich in calcium, iron, fiber and vitamin A.

Healthy Fats

Our bodies need the essential amino acids to function properly. They can be obtained from nuts and seeds, avocado, soya products and other plant based foods.

A plant based diet is known to provide cardiovascular and health benefits to many people are concerned about cancer. They also provide anti-inflammatory properties that discourage development of many illnesses and diseases. Many diseases arise from inflammatory factors within the system. Eating plant power foods is the best thing you can do to your overall health. They will boost your immune system and get rid of toxins from your body.

There are certain plant based foods which you can take to derive optimal health benefits.

These include organically grown

- whole grains
- fruits
- vegetables
- healthy fats
- nuts and seeds
- tubers
- legumes

There are people who assume that, moving from a meat-based diet to a plant based diet will tie them up into a dull lifestyle. This is far from the truth. A plant based diet is so delicious that you will not miss a thing about meat. Just in case you do miss it, you can add soy products like tofu and tempeh in your diet.

When you get a flare-up from meat based foods and processed foods, stop eating them altogether and know that it is your body talking to you. However, you don't have to wait until you fall sick to start taking Plant Power Foods. Start taking them today if you want to live a healthy life full of vibrant energy. Many people are allergic to milk, cheese, cream, wheat and wheat products, meat and eggs and they fall sick without changing their diet.

2: Breakfast Recipes

Recipe 1:

Gluten-free Banana Bread

This low-gluten vegetarian bread is prepared with little or no sugar. You can ice the bread if you like.

Time: 30 minutes (10 for preparation, 20 for baking)

Ingredients:

- 4-6 ripe bananas
- 2 cups rice floor
- 1 cup ground oats
- 1½ cups of water
- ¼ cup honey or ½ cup natural sugar
- 4 tablespoons coconut oil
- 1 tablespoon baking soda
- 1 teaspoon vanilla extract
- 1 teaspoon salt

Optional

- ¼ cup dry raisins or berries
- ¼ cup ground nuts

- cardamom, cinnamon and cloves

Instructions:

Pre-heat the oven at 350 degrees F or 180 degrees C.

Start by mixing rice flour, oats and baking soda together in a mixing bowl and ensure that the mixture does not have clumps. You can do this with your hand or you can sieve it. Keep the mixture aside.

Take a saucepan and add to it water, honey, oil, salt, vanilla extract and the spices. Warm this mixture for 5-10 minutes in warm temperatures. Ensure that all these ingredients have dissolved especially if you are using natural sugar. Add the dried fruits and nuts. When cooled, add it to the dry mixture and mix it thoroughly.

Mash the ripe bananas until there are no clumps and add them to the mixture in the mixing bowl.

Use the coconut oil to grease the banana bread baking tins and pour the mixture into about 3-4 tins. Spread it so the breads are thin but not so thin.

Bake until you can see a few cracks on the bread and this should be about 20 minutes or more. The time the bread bakes depends on the thickness. Remove from oven once ready and let the breads cool.

Recipe 2:

Sweet Potato and Oatmeal Breakfast

Tubers can be a great addition to your breakfast recipe whether they are sweet potatoes, potatoes, arrow-roots or yams. Add sweet potatoes to your oatmeal and start your day with added energy.

Serves: 3

Ingredients:

- 1 cup sweet potatoes, peeled and chopped
- 2 cups coconut milk, unsweetened
- ½ cup oats, cut
- ½ teaspoon of cinnamon, ground
- maple agape or brown sugar to sweeten

Preparation

Peel and chop yellow, white or purple sweet potatoes (the color depends on your preference).

Cook them with the oats slowly in low heat until they are ready. Mash them with a potato masher or fork. Serve in 2 bowls and add coconut milk and maple agape or brown sugar to sweeten your breakfast. Even kids love this breakfast.

You can add a pinch of nutmeg and cloves if you like.

Recipe 3:

Apple and Cucumber Salad

Take whole fruits and veggies for breakfast or whip up a salad or juice to start your day with a boost of energy.

- 1 cucumber, sliced
- 1 apple, cored
- ½ lemon, squeezed juice

Preparation

Start your day by slicing the cucumber and cored apple and adding freshly squeezed lemon juice. Mix them into a refreshing and crispy fruit salad which you will enjoy.

Recipe 4:

Brown Rice and Squash Breakfast

Cooked brown rice can be taken when you are not taking oatmeal. They make a great breakfast also. You can heat up some of the dinner leftovers in the morning and use them to enrich your breakfast.

Serves: 4

Ingredients:

- ½ medium squash or yams
- 2 cups water
- 1 cup brown rice
- ½ Tablespoon fresh sage, chopped
- 1 Tablespoon shallots, minced
- 3 Tablespoon vegetable oil or coconut oil
- salt to taste

Preparation

Preheat the oven at 400 degrees F. Cut the squash into two and remove the seeds. Apply some oil on the cut sides and put the squash halves on a baking sheet upside down. Bake for 45 minutes and use a fork to check if it is cooked by pricking. Remove from oven and wait until they are warm. Cut into cubes with or without the skin.

Put the water in the saucepan and put on medium heat. Add the rice when the water boils and cover the saucepan. Bring it to a boil and lower the heat. Simmer until it is cooked. Blend the shallots, sage and salt. Take a saucepan and add the oil. Cook on low heat. Add the rice and shallots, sage and salt mixture and stir. Cook the rice for about 1 minute stirring consistently. Remove from heat and mix with the squash. Serve.

Recipe 5:

Gluten Free, Sugar Free, Cranberry and Kale Smoothie

Berries have antibacterial and antiviral properties and that is why they should be consumed regularly throughout the year. Strawberries, blueberries, blackberries, raspberries and cranberries have also anti-inflammatory benefits. Cranberries are usually overlooked but they are a super-food that you can enjoy. They are inexpensive and you should add them to your diet.

They can perform the following functions in the body:

- cancer prevention and destroying tumor cell growth
- cleansing the urinary tract
- promoting detoxification of the liver

Plant based foods provide us with anti-cancer prevention benefits. Cranberries and the other berry family are antioxidants that are known to fight cancer cell growth, boost the immune system and fight illnesses and diseases when they are consumed regularly. Cranberries cleanse the liver and blood of toxins which cause diseases.

Ingredients:

- 2 cups fresh cranberries, organic
- 4 leaves kale, without the hard stem
- 1 banana, organic
- 1 ½ cups non-dairy milk or coconut water
- 1 teaspoon cinnamon, ground
- 2 dates or other natural sweetener

Preparation

Remove the hard stem of the kale leaves and cut them roughly with your hands. Put them in the blender and add all the other ingredients and puree until smooth. Serve into a large glass and enjoy.

Recipe 6:

Cranberry and Pumpkin Bread

Serves: 10

Ingredients:

- 1.75 oz cranberries
- 2 cups pumpkin mash or puree
- 2 teaspoon pumpkin pie spice
- 1 ½ whole-meal wheat flour
- 1 teaspoon baking powder
- ½ cup maple syrup
- 1 teaspoon vanilla extract
- 2 Tablespoons non-dairy milk
- natural peanut butter

Method

Preheat the oven at 35o degrees F or 180 degrees C.

To make this loaf, you need to grease a loaf tin and keep it aside then sieve all the dry ingredients in a mixing bowl. Use your hands to roll on the other ingredients and mix them thoroughly except maple syrup and butter which you will use while serving. Spread the mixture and bake the bread. Cut into slices and spread the butter on the slices sprinkling with maple syrup. You can keep the bread for 3 days out of the fridge or more days in the fridge.

Recipe 7:

Easy to Make Power Breakfast

If you are looking for an easy to make breakfast to kick off your day then you are at the right place.

Ingredients:

- 1 Tablespoon of dried fruits like cranberries, raisins, apricots
- 1 Tablespoon of seeds like pumpkin seeds, flaxseed, linseed
- 1 Tablespoon of mixed nuts such as hazelnuts, almonds, brazil nuts
- 2 Tablespoons of wheat germ in your oatmeal porridge using non-daily milk

Mix the ingredients in a bowl and enjoy.

3: Dips and Appetizers

You can add or lessen the ingredients in the following recipes to get what you like.

Recipe 8:

Fresh Homemade Salsa and Sauce

This vegetarian salsa and sauce looks so colorful and it tastes yummy. It is a good idea when you grow tomatoes in the garden because you can have plenty of them during summer.

Serving: 1 jar

Ingredients:

- 3 pounds ripe tomatoes (chopped)
- 2 small jalapeno peppers (chopped)
- 1 clove garlic (minced)
- ½ peeled onion (chopped)
- ½ teaspoon red wine vinegar
- ½ lime or lemon freshly squeezed juice
- 1 handful of cilantro
- pinch of salt and pepper as seasoning

Instructions:

Mix the chopped tomatoes, jalapeno peppers and onions in a bowl. Add them and the other ingredients into the food processor and pulse until it is the texture you like. You can have it smooth or coarse depending on your consistency preference.

Serve the salsa with veggies, chips or top it on your meals especially Mexican dishes, it will all taste delicious.

You can keep it in the fridge in an air tight container or in a glass jar for 1 week. After this, the taste starts changing. You can cook the salsa and cool it then can it, so it can stay longer.

You can lower the ingredients to make less salsa. Those who like chunky tomatoes in their salsa can pulse some of them first and add chucks of tomatoes later. Grow organic tomatoes in your garden and use them to make natural healthy salsa and sauce

Recipe 9:

Pomegranates and Avocado Salsa

The pomegranate and avocado salsa is a favorite to so many people of different ages. Even kids love the sweetness that comes with pomegranate seeds and they are also easy to add to your meals when you are on the go. You can have pomegranates with avocado, pancakes, yogurt, salsas, salads and many other dishes. You can eat the delicious pomegranates and avocado salsa to compliment chips, burgers, tacos and other dishes.

Serving: 2 cups

Ingredients:

- ½ cup pomegranate seeds (arils)
- 1 large avocado, diced
- 1 small shallot, chopped
- 1 teaspoon cilantro, chopped
- 1 lime, freshly squeezed juice
- pinch of salt
- pepper to taste

Optional

- 1 diced jalapeno to make it spicy

Instructions:

Mix shallot, cilantro, avocado and lime juice together in a mixture bowl. Add pomegranate seeds, salt and pepper as seasoning and mix. If you like spicy salsa, then add diced jalapeno. Serve in 2 cups and enjoy.

Recipe 10:

Tomato and Onion Salsa

Serving: 4-6

Ingredients:

- 1 cup diced tomato
- ½ cup diced onions
- ¼ cup fresh lime juice
- 20 sprigs minced cilantro
- ½ teaspoon salt

Optional

- ¼ teaspoon black pepper
- ½ teaspoon cayenne pepper

Instructions:

Put the onions in a bowl and add the fresh lime juice. Wait for 5 minutes to add tomatoes, cilantro, salt and pepper. You can season the salsa with other types of pepper to season it. Cover and store in the fridge for 30 minutes and serve.

Recipe 11:

Fresh Tomato and Salsa

Serves: 6

Ingredients:

- 4 large fresh tomatoes, chopped
- 1 cup onion, diced
- 4 garlic cloves, minced
- 1 fresh green bell pepper, minced
- 4 teaspoons jalapeno pepper without the seeds, diced
- ¼ cup cilantro, minced
- 2 teaspoons fresh lime juice, squeezed
- ½ cumin, ground
- ½ Kosher salt
- ½ pepper

Place the ingredients in a bowl and mix thoroughly. Keep in the fridge for 24 hours and serve. You will like the flavor. If you like the salsa spicy, then dice the jalapeno together with the seeds.

Recipe 12:

Pomegranate and Apple Appetizer

Serves: 4-6

Ingredients:

- 1 full pomegranate, seeds
- 2 cups of pomegranate juice
- 1 large chopped apple
- ¼ cup chopped fresh mint,
- 1 bottle pure water
- some crushed ice

Instructions:

Mix pomegranate seeds and juice, chopped apple and some of the mint together in a mixture bowl. Put the crushed ice and water in bowls and serve the mixture over the ice. Garnish with some mint.

Recipe 13:

Fleshly Prepared Salsa

Serves: 4-6

Ingredients:

- ½ cup diced onions
- 1 cup diced tomato
- ¼ cup fresh lime juice

- 20 sprigs minced cilantro
- ½ teaspoon salt

Optional

- ¼ teaspoon black pepper
- ½ teaspoon cayenne pepper

Instructions:

Put the onions in a bowl and add the fresh lime juice. Wait for 5 minutes to add tomatoes, cilantro, salt and pepper. You can season the salsa with other types of pepper to make it taste better. Cover and store in the fridge for 30 minutes and serve.

4: Quick Meals and Snacks

Recipe 14:

Vegan Tempeh Sandwich

This is a gluten-free, dairy free vegan sandwich which is rich in nutrients. You can use tempeh to make a vegan sandwich

Serves: 2

Ingredients:

- 1 block of tempeh, cut into 8 rectangular pieces
- 4 pieces gluten-free bread
- 1 tablespoon canola oil
- 2 tablespoons vegan butter
- 2 tablespoons balsamic vinegar
- 2 tablespoons apple cider vinegar, raw
- 2 tablespoons extra-virgin olive oil
- 2 tablespoons gluten-free tamari
- 2 tablespoons water
- 2 cloves garlic, minced
- 1 tablespoons gluten-free veggie sauce
- 1 bay leaf, crumbled

- 1 teaspoon of each of the following-paprika, onion powder, dried coriander, smoked paprika and dried mustard

Dressing

- 2 tablespoons ketchup
- 1 teaspoon gluten-free vegan sauce
- 1/3 cup mayonnaise
- 1 tablespoon horse radish, prepared
- Kosher salt to taste
- pepper to taste

Preparation

1. Combine balsamic vinegar, apple cider vinegar, extra-virgin olive oil, gluten-free tamari, water, garlic, gluten-free veggie sauce, bay leaf, paprika, onion powder, dried coriander, smoked paprika and dried mustard together in a bowl and stir into a rich mixture.

2. Cut the tempeh into 8 pieces and add it to the mixture and let it marinate for 1 hour. Prepare the dressing in the meantime.

3. Pre-heat the grill at medium-high. Put the extra-virgin olive oil on the grill pan and cook the tempeh pieces until they brown and soften on both sides which takes about 4 minutes for each side. Remove them from the pan and set them aside.

4. Take a skillet and heat it on medium-high heat and as it heats-up apply butter on one side of each slice of bread. Place the buttered sides to cook on the skillet until they become golden brown. Place the slices on a flat surface with the golden brown sides facing upwards. Spread the dressing on the 1st slice and place 4 pieces of tempeh on top of the dressing.

5. Place the 2nd slice of bread on top of the sandwich with the golden brown side facing downwards to make the first sandwich. Prepare another sandwich the same way using the 3rd and 4th slices and the remaining ingredients.

6. Put each of the sandwiches on the slitter at medium-high heat and brown both sides of each of the two sandwiches and turn them

gently. Serve the sandwiches while they are hot.

Recipe 15:

Avocado Guacamole Recipe

Serves: 8

Ready in: 10 minutes

Ingredients:

- 4 large ripe avocadoes 8 oz each, seeded and peeled
- 1Tbs. fresh lemon juice, squeezed
- ½ small sweet onion, diced
- 1 ripe tomato, diced
- pepper and salt to taste

Preparation

Mash the avocadoes with fresh lemon juice and leave some chunks so it is not smooth, then add all the other ingredient and mix gently. Serve in bowls. You can add any of the following to make the flavor you like jalapeno, cilantro, onion, tomato, garlic or more pepper and salt.

Recipe 16:

Avocado, Tomato, Lettuce with Cucumber Sandwich

Serves: 4

Ingredients:

- 8 slices of whole bread, toasted
- 1 large ripe avocado, sliced
- 1 large tomato, thinly sliced
- 4 lettuce leaves
- 2 Tbs. non-dairy mayonnaise

Preparation

Spread the mayonnaise on 4 slices of bread and put lettuce leaves on the slices. Top with slices of avocado, tomatoes and cucumber. Cover with the remaining 4 slices of bread. Cut each sandwich into 2 halves diagonally with a knife and serve.

Recipe 17:

Vegetarian Rice Noodle Soup

Serves: 6

Ingredients:

- 8oz. dried vermicelli noodle
- 1 onion
- ¼ tsp. black pepper
- ¼ chopped cilantro
- ¼ cup fresh mushroom
- 1 Tbs. vegetable oil
- 2 cloves garlic
- ¼ red pepper
- 2 tsp. salt
- Lime wedges
- Seasonal vegetable of your choice
- Chopped jalapeno pepper

Place noodle in a large bowl. Add 6 cup boiling water to the noodle. Wait 2 minutes. Drain and rinse with cold water. Using a wok, fry the onions for few minutes until cooked. Add garlic and stir for about 45 seconds. Add salt and pepper along with 6 cups of boiling water. Let it simmer for 3 minutes. Add peppers, mushrooms and herbs. Let is simmer for 3-4 minutes.

Preparation

Pour rice noodles into a bowl. Add broth on top. Garnish the meal with lime wedges and jalapeno pepper. Serve. Enjoy

Recipe 18:

Zucchini Avocado Soup with Cucumber Salsa

Serves: 4

Ingredients:

- 2 medium zucchini, chopped
- 1 large cucumber, peeled and seeded
- 1 can vegetable broth 14 oz
- 1 large avocado, peeled and diced
- 1 Tbs. fresh cilantro, chopped
- ½ cup green onions, chopped
- 3 Tbs. lime juice, squeezed ½ t salt
- ¼ t cumin, ground
- ¾ cup vegan milk

Take a saucepan and put the vegetable broth, half of the green onions and zucchini and allow the ingredients to boil. Cover with a lid and simmer for 7 min ensuring that the zucchini pieces are tender. Remove from heat and keep aside to cool.

Put the other half of green onions on a skillet or saucepan with cilantro, 1 Tbs. lime juice, ¼ teaspoon salt and cucumber. Mix and keep aside as cucumber salsa.

Take a blender and put the zucchini mixture, vegan milk, ¼ teaspoon of salt, cumin and 2 Tbs. of fresh lime juice in and puree until the soup is smooth. Serve hot or chilly with Cucumber salsa

Recipe 19:

Banana and Rice Snacks

Ingredients:

- 3 organic bananas, mashed
- 2 cups brown rice
- 1 cup vegan milk like soy milk or almond milk
- ¼ cup flaxseeds, ground
- ½ cup arrowroot flour, ground
- ¾ cup maple syrup
- ¼ cup coconut oil
- 1 Tbs. soy sauce
- 1 Tbs. rice vinegar

- 1 tsp baking powder
- ½ tsp baking soda
- salt to taste

Optional

- ½ tsp cinnamon
- 1 tsp cardamon

Preparation

Preheat the oven at 350 degrees F.

Mix all the dry ingredients together in a bowl and sift them. Mash the organic bananas and add maple syrup or agape syrup and coconut oil. Use your hands to make a hollow in the middle of the dry ingredients and put the wet mixture in the center. Mix all the ingredients by hand. Oil a baking sheet or cookie sheet and use your hands to create some cookies. Bake for 20 minutes. Scones should be organic in shape and drop like a cookie.

Recipe 20:
Beet Cleansing Soup

- 2 celery stalks, chopped

- 2 beet green stalks, chopped
- 1 cup cilantro, chopped
- 1 lime, peeled, seeded and chopped
- 2 cloves of garlic, minced
- 2 Tbs. olive oil
- some apple cider vinegar
- cayenne pepper
- 4 cups water

Preparation

Chop all veggies into medium-size country style pieces. In a pot over medium heat, sauté garlic in olive oil. Add celery and stir until the color brightens. Add beet greens, cilantro, lime, cayenne pepper and filtered water. Before serving, add a splash of apple cider vinegar. Simmer on low heat for 30 minutes. Serve.

5: Main Dish, Stews and Soups Recipes

Any of the following dishes, stews and soups can be served with whole grains like brown rice, whole wheat bread, chips, pancakes, chips and anything else that your taste buds. Most of them can be used as filings to make a yummy meal for yourself, your kids or for guests.

Recipe 21:

Pomegranate, Coconut and Sweet Potatoes

This tropical recipe is rich in nutrients.

Serving: 4

- 4 medium sweet potatoes, washed
- 2 tablespoons cilantro, chopped
- 1 cup pomegranate seeds
- ½ cup coconut milk, light
- ¼ toasted coconut flakes, unsweetened
- pieces of lime wedges
- Salt to taste

Instructions:

Pre-heat the oven at 400 degrees F.

Arrange the sweet potatoes on a baking sheet and prick them with a fork to ensure that they get cooked inside. Bake them for 45 minutes or until they become tender. Remove them from oven and let them cool slightly. If you let them cool completely they might harden.

Peel the top of the potatoes and mash each one of them. Use a fork to mash. Mix the cilantro, pomegranate seeds, coconut flakes and coconut milk in a bowl. Add salt to taste. Divide the mixture into 4 portions and put as topping on the mashed sweet potatoes. Serve with the pieces of lime wedges.

Recipe 22:

Gluten-Free Black-Eyed Peas and Collard Soup

Celery is a rich source of antioxidants such as Vitamin C, Vitamin B6, Vitamin K, calcium, iron, Riboflavin, low-calorific dietary fiber, magnesium, manganese and phosphorous. Collard greens are a good source of calcium.

Serves: 6

Ready by: 45 minutes

Ingredients:

- 2 cups black-eyed dry peas, rinsed
- 1 pound collard greens, chopped without the stem
- 2 medium onions, diced
- 2 stems of celery, diced
- 1 green bell pepper, diced
- 3 cloves garlic, diced
- 6 cups water

Preparation

Sort the black-eyed peas and boil them with water in a cooking pot until they are soft. Remove stem of collard greens and chop them.

Spray the pressure cooker or pot with olive oil. Heat it and put the onions. Sauté the onions until they are light brown then add green pepper, garlic and celery for 3 minutes while stirring.

Recipe 23:

Black Bean Soup

Serves: 2

Ready by: 45 minutes

Ingredients:

- 1 tin black beans 15oz, drained and rinsed
- 1 medium onion, chopped
- 1 teaspoon cumin, ground
- 1 teaspoon chili powder
- 1 ½ vegetable broth
- 2 teaspoons fresh lime juice
- ¼ or ½ salsa of your choice

Garnish

- 2 tablespoon cilantro, chopped
- 1 green onion, chopped

Optional

- Cayenne pepper or hot sauce

Preparation

Put some water or vegetable broth in a skillet then add onions and sauté for 3 minutes in high heat. Combine with cumin and curry powder while you stir. Add the black beans, your favorite salsa and the remaining vegetable broth. When it boils simmer for 10 minutes in low heat. Remove from heat and add the lime juice.

Divide the mixture into 2 halves. Put one-half in the blender. Blend until it is smooth and mix it with the other half. Garnish the soup with cilantro and green onions. Add cayenne or hot sauce if you like.

Recipe 24:

Spinach Couscous and Chickpea with Cashews

Serves: 4-6

Ingredients:

- 1 cup whole wheat couscous
- 2 cups fresh baby spinach
- 3 garlic cloves, finely chopped
- 2 Tablespoons olive oil
- 1 can organic tomatoes 28 oz, diced
- 1 can chickpeas 14oz (or kidney peas or navy beans), drained and rinsed
- 1 medium onion, chopped
- 1 teaspoons cumin, ground
- 1 teaspoon coriander, ground
- 1 teaspoon black pepper

- ½ lemon juice
- ¼ cup toasted cashews
- water
- salt to taste

Preparation

Take a small pot and put water in it. Boil it and remove from heat and add couscous then cover with a lid for 5 minutes and remove from water, setting it aside.

Put oil on a saucepan over medium heat and add onions and garlic. Sauté until they are lightly brown and then add coriander, garlic, cumin and salt to the mixture. Mix in the tomatoes and lower the heat. Simmer for 10 minutes then add the spinach and chickpeas stirring consistently. Taste and see if there will be need to add the seasonings. When it is cooked remove from heat. Serve the couscous in bowls then put the spinach and chickpea stew on top Garnish with roasted cashew nuts.

Recipe 25:

Black Bean with Rice and Salsa

Serves: 2

Ready by: 25 minutes

Ingredients:

- 1 tin black beans 15oz, un-drained
- 1 medium onion, chopped
- 1 can tomatoes14.5 oz, stewed
- 1 ½ cups uncooked brown rice, instant
- 1 tablespoon of vegetable oil
- 1 teaspoon of dry oregano
- ½ teaspoon of garlic powder

Preparation

Put vegetable oil in a large saucepan and heat on medium heat. Add onions and sauté for 3 minutes until they become tender. Combine with dry oregano, tomatoes, un-drained beans and garlic powder while you stir. Put on high heat and let it boil and then add the uncooked rice and stir. Cover the mixture and simmer until the rice is properly cooked which is about 5 minutes. Remove from heat and wait for 5 minutes to serve.

Recipe 26:

Spinach Chickpea and Tofu Curry

Serves: 4

Ready by: 20 minutes

Ingredients:

- 1 can chickpeas 15 oz, drained and rinsed
- 1 packaged tofu 12 oz, cubed
- 1 medium onion, diced
- 1 bunch of spinach, with stems removed
- 1 tablespoon curry paste
- 1 teaspoon basil, dried
- 1 can corn
- ½ teaspoon garlic powder
- salt to taste
- pepper, ground

Preparation

Use a large skillet or wok to cook this curry. Put the vegetable oil on the wok and heat it on medium heat. Add the onions and sauté them until they are light brown then add corn and the curry powder and keep stirring as it cooks for 5 minutes. Put salt, garlic and pepper and stir consistently.

Add the beans and tofu and lay the spinach on top of the mixture. Cover with a lid and when the spinach is cooked remove the wok from the heat. Stir in the dried basil and serve.

Recipe 27:

Mushrooms and Broccoli with Tofu

Serves: 4

Ready in: 20 minutes

Ingredients:

- 5 mushrooms, fresh and chopped
- 1 small broccoli, chopped into florets
- 1 pound Tofu, cubed
- 2 Tbs. soy sauce
- 1 Tbs. peanut oil
- 1 small bell pepper, sliced
- 2 Tbs. vinegar
- ½ cup peanut butter
- ½ cup water

- pinch of cayenne pepper
- salt to taste

Put oil on a skillet and put over medium-high heat, sauté the chopped mushrooms, cubed tofu, bell pepper slices and broccoli for 5 minutes.

Mix all the other ingredients in a mixing bowl and add to the cooking. Mix consistently until ready. Serve.

Recipe 28:

Ginger and Vegetable Stir-Fry

In this stir-fry, you can substitute any vegetables with the ones in season. You can add the ingredients such as ginger and garlic to give it more.

You can add tofu and if you are not for crunchy vegetables, you may add some water and cook them longer or just lower the heat.

Serves: 6

Ready by: 40 minutes

Ingredients:

- 1 large onion, chopped
- green beans halved
- ¾ cup carrots, chopped
- 1 tablespoon of corn starch
- 2 cloves garlic, crushed
- 2 teaspoon ginger, ground
- ¼ cup vegetable oil
- 1 small broccoli, florets
- ½ cup snow peas
- 2 tablespoons soy sauce
- 2 tablespoons water
- ½ tablespoons salt

Preparation

Combine ginger, garlic, corn start and a little vegetable oil and mix them until the corn starch dissolves completely. Add the snow peas, carrots, green beans and broccoli and mix.

Use a wok or large skillet to heat the other vegetable oil on medium heat. Cook the mixture for 2 minutes and while you keep on stirring otherwise the food may burn. Add the soy sauce and stir then add the water. Stir in the onions, ginger and water until the vegetables are cooked. The curry will be crunch but if you want it to be soft and tender, you can cook for a longer time or at low heat.

Recipe 29:

Celery Fries

Celery has anti-inflammatory health benefits, making it one of the healthiest vegetables available today. You can use celery in salads, stews, soups and broths or stir-fry it.

Serves: 6

Preparation time: 15 min

Cooking time: 5 min

Ready in 20 minutes

Ingredients:

- 2 Tablespoons canola oil
- 4 cups of shaped celery stalks
- 3 dry Chile peppers
- 2 Tablespoons of sesame oil
- 2 Tablespoons of soy sauce

Preparation

Cut off the root of the celery and then cut the stalks in thin long shapes for frying. Put canola oil and Chile peppers on a frying pan and heat for 90 seconds. Fry the celery in the oil and if you like, you can add sesame oil. Stir-fry the celery and add soy sauce after 3 minutes of frying and fry for another 1 minute. Serve while hot with brown rice or any other dish.

Recipe 30:

Spinach, Chickpea and Tofu Curry

Serves: 4

Ready by: 20 minutes

Ingredients:

- 1 can black beans 15 oz, drained and rinsed
- 8 oz cherry tomatoes , halved
- 1 can tofu
- 1 jalapeno, diced finely
- 1 bunch of spinach, with stems removed
- 1 tablespoon curry paste
- 1 teaspoon basil, dried
- 1 can of corn
- ½ teaspoon garlic powder

- salt to taste
- pepper, ground

Preparation

Use a large skillet or wok to cook this curry. Put the vegetable oil on the wok and heat it on medium heat. Add the onions and sauté them until they are light brown then add corn and the curry powder and keep stirring as it cooks for 5 minutes. Put salt, garlic and pepper and stir consistently.

Add the beans and tofu and lay the spinach on top of the mixture. Cover with a lid and when the spinach is cooked remove the wok from the heat. Stir in the dried basil and serve.

Recipe 31:

Spicy Onions with Tempeh

Tempeh is a plant power soy bean product that has been fermented and is a good source of protein. You can purchase it in most grocery stores and health stores. Each serving of tempeh should give you 15-20 grams of protein.

Ingredients:

- 1 cup organic Tempeh
- 2 medium onions
- 1green chili, chopped
- 1 green chili, sliced thinly
- 1 Tablespoon canola oil
- 1 Tablespoon coriander leaves, chopped
- 1 Tablespoon mint leaves, chopped
- 1 small ginger piece, chopped
- 1 teaspoon cumin seeds
- 1 teaspoon coriander seeds
- 1 teaspoon vegetable oil or vegan butter
- 1 teaspoon fresh lime juice, squeezed
- ½ teaspoon turmeric powder
- ½ raw sugar
- salt to taste
- water

Instructions:

Cut one of the green chili thinly and chop the other one. Cut the onions into rounded rings. Place a saucepan on medium heat and put half of the canola oil and add onion. Sauté them and add the sliced green chili and cilantro leaves and stir them for 3 minutes. Remove them from the heat and keep them aside.

You can use the same saucepan to cook the following ingredients. Take the remaining canola oil, onions and chopped green chili and add them on the saucepan and cook on medium heat. Add coriander, turmeric and cumin and keep stirring until the onions turn golden brown. Mix in mint leaves and the ginger and cook for 1 minute. Add lemon juice, veggie butter, pepper and salt and stir.

Place the chopped tempeh pieces on the mixture and mix with the cooked ingredients. Cover the saucepan and cook for 20 to 25 minutes depending on the size of the tempeh pieces. Add water and let the curry boil for another 10 minutes to thicken the puree. Serve while it is hot and place the onion, green chili and cilantro mixture which you had kept aside on top. You can eat the curry with bread, rice or another dish.

You can add Fenugreek seeds with the other spices.

Recipe 32:

Mushrooms and Barley with Onions

Serves: 4-6

Ingredients:

- 10 oz white mushrooms
- 1 cup barley
- 3 or 3 ½ cups vegetable broth or water
- 3 cloves of garlic, minced
- 2 large onions, thinly sliced
- 2 Tablespoons olive oil
- 2 Teaspoons fresh dill or parsley, minced
- pepper and salt

Instructions:

Put 3 cups of vegetable broth or water in a pot or saucepan and boil on medium-high then cover with a lid and simmer for 40 minutes in low heat.

Take a skillet and put the oil. Add the onions and sauté them until they become translucent. Mix in the garlic until the onions become lightly brown. Add the white mushrooms and stir. Put ¼ cup water and cover, let them cook on medium heat until they are ready which should be about 8 minutes.

Add the cooked barley to the mushrooms and continue stirring. Add the dill or parsley, peeper and salt and stir thoroughly. Use freshly ground pepper and either dill or parsley depending on what you prefer. Cook for 3 minutes and serve.

Recipe 33:

Zucchini, Shallot and Avocado

Serves: 4

Ingredients:

- 3 zucchinis, sliced into long strips lengthwise
- 1 ripe avocado chopped into chunks, peeled and seeded
- 2 Tbs. olive oil
- 2 tsp. garlic, finely chopped
- 1 small shallot, finely chopped
- 1 ½ lime, squeeze juice
- ½ bell pepper, squared
- 1 Tbs. lemon rind, grated
- ½ thyme leaves, fresh

Instructions:

Put oil on a non-stick skillet on medium-high and add olive oil, thyme and garlic and then sauté for 3 minutes. Add zucchini, lemon rind and pepper then cook for 5 minutes. Remember to stir regular. Mix in the freshly squeezed lemon juice and avocado and stir gently as you cook for another 2 minutes. Serve.

Recipe 34:

Sweet Potato Soup with Great Flavor

Serves: 4

Preparation Time: 15 min

Cooking Time: 20 min

Ready by: 35 minutes

Ingredients:

- 1 peeled sweet potato, skinned and chopped
- 1 onion, chopped thinly
- 4 cups spinach, chopped
- 3 garlic cloves, minced
- ½ teaspoon garam masala
- ½ teaspoon turmeric powder
- 2 cups vegetable broth

- 2 red pepper flakes
- water
- salt to taste

Instructions:

Chop the skinned sweet potatoes into cubes and keep it aside. Place a saucepan on medium heat and put some water into it. Add onions and garlic, sauté them for 1 minute then mix in the red pepper flakes and keep stirring until the water dries up. Put the lentils, turmeric, garam masala, vegetable broth and let it boil. Simmer and cook for 5 minutes on low heat.

Toss in the cubed sweet potatoes and simmer when the mixture boils until the lentils are soft and the potatoes are tender. Check the potatoes by pricking them with a fork. You can add more vegetable broth or water if either the potatoes or lentils are not cooked.

Add the spinach and some garam masala if you like adding some and keep stirring until the spinach softens. Sprinkle the salt to taste and stir.

Recipe 35:

Tasty Pea Soup

This soup is colorful and is full of flavor.

Serves: 8

Ingredients:

- 1 onion, chopped
- 2 cups of split green peas
- 8 cups vegetable stock, low-sodium
- ¼ cup of barley
- 2 chopped carrots
- 2 chopped potatoes
- 2 chopped celery stalks
- 2 bay leaves
- 2 tablespoons parsley flakes
- 1 teaspoon of celery seeds
- 1 teaspoon of paprika
- 1 teaspoon of basil
- White pepper, red pepper and salt to taste

Instructions:

Start by putting the split beans, vegetable stock and barley in a pot and allowing it to boil while covered. Lower the heat, add celery seeds and bay leaves and let the ingredients boil for half an hour. Add all the other ingredients and boil in low heat for another 1 hour to make the soup thick and flavorful.

You can serve with brown rice, pasta or baked potatoes.

Recipe 36:

White Beans, Carrots Vegetable Soup

Serves: 4-6

Preparation Time: 20 min

Cooking Time: 30 min

Ready in: 50 minutes

Ingredients:

- 1 onion, chopped
- 2 cans navy beans 15 oz, drained and rinsed
- 2 cups chopped kale or spinach, without the stem
- 4 cups vegetable broth
- 2 cup of small size whole wheat macaroni, uncooked

- 1 sliced carrots
- 1 can red tomatoes, fire roasted
- 1 lime, squeezed juice
- 4 cups water
- red pepper and salt to taste

Instructions:

Use a large saucepan and put some little vegetable broth to cook the carrots and onions on medium-high, until cooked. You can add more vegetable broth if the carrots have not softened. This should take about 5 minutes to cook. Add water, the remaining vegetable broth, beans and the fire roasted tomatoes. Cover the saucepan and bring to the boil. Simmer and cook for 20 minutes.

In order to thicken the soup, you can use a bean masher to mash some of the food or blend it in a blender. Put the macaroni and cook for 2 minutes, then add kale or spinach and cook an additional 5 minutes.

Remove the soup from the heat and add salt, pepper and lime juice.

Recipe 37:

Chickpea and Sweet Potato Cakes with Avocado

Preparation time: 40 minutes

To serve: 4

Ingredients:

- 1 ¾ cups grated sweet potatoes
- 1 tin drained and cleaned chickpeas (15 oz)
- 1 pound broccoli, chopped in florets
- 2 ½ tablespoon olive oil
- 1 tablespoon freshly squeezed lemon juice
- ½ cup yellow onion, chopped
- 6 crushed garlic cloves
- 1 cup chopped tomatoes
- ½ cup breadcrumbs
- 1 peeled and chopped avocado
- 2 teaspoons grated or finely cut lemon rind
- 1/8 teaspoon black pepper (freshly ground)
- ½ cup long and thinly cut red onions
- ½ cup non-dairy milk
- Pinch of salt to taste

Pre-heat the oven to 400 degrees F.

Take a pan and put 1 tablespoon of oil. Add yellow onion and garlic to the pan and sauté them for 3 minutes. Add the sweet potatoes, salt and pepper and sauté for another 2 minutes. Pour the sweet potato mixture, breadcrumbs, non-dairy milk, chickpeas and 1 ½ lemon juice into a food processor and work on it until it has a coarse texture.

Divide the mixture into 4 equal portions and shape them in rounds flattening them a bit with your hands. Roll them on breadcrumbs and bake. Serve the sweet potato cakes and chickpea cakes with avocado.

Recipe 38:

Tofu-Fry with Broccoli

Serves: 2

Ingredients:

- 16 oz firm tofu, thawed
- 2 Tbs. garlic, finely minced
- 1 cup corn starch
- 1Tbs.soy sauce

- 1 Tbs. ginger, shredded
- 1 Tbs. white vinegar
- 1 Tbs. agave syrup
- 1 cup water enough vegetable oil (for frying)
- 1 cup broccoli, cut in florets

Preparation

You can substitute agape syrup with maple syrup or vegan sugar

Cut the tofu in cubes and toss them in closed container with corn starch (as much as you desire). In a small saucepan, put the oil on medium heat and fry some of the tofu turning them on the other side until they are lightly brown. Fry the remaining tofu the same way. In the meantime steam the broccoli.

Sauce

To make sauce, sauté the ginger, garlic and red peppers, in a saucepan with oil, over medium heat, while stirring regularly. Add agape syrup or vegan sugar, vinegar, soy sauce and water while ensuring that the sugar dissolves completely. If you want to thicken the sauce mix 1 Tablespoons of cold water and 1 teaspoon of corn oil and stir it in the sauce mixture. Bring it to a boil for a few minutes. Remove from the heat and let it cool. Mix with tofu.

Serve the tofu with steamed broccoli and brown rice.

Recipe 39:

Eggplant Soup

Ingredients:

- 1 large or 1 ½ pounds eggplant, sliced in halves
- 3 tomatoes, sliced in halves
- 4 cups vegetable broth
- 1 onion, halved
- 6 garlic cloves, peeled
- 2 Tablespoons vegetable oil
- 1 Tablespoon thyme, chopped
- pepper and salt to taste

Preparation

Preheat the oven at 400 degrees F.

Place eggplants, onions, garlic and tomatoes on a baking sheet and sprinkle with vegetable oil. Put them in the oven to roast for 45 minutes. Remove them from the oven when the vegetables have become tender and lightly brown with spots. Peel the eggplants and place them in a saucepan, add thyme and the other roasted vegetables and the vegetable broth. Bring to a boil and simmer for 45 minutes.

Remove from heat and let the vegetables cool. Put in a blender and puree until smooth. Return the soup back to the saucepan and add more vegetable broth if you like it thinner. Add pepper and salt to taste. Serve in bowls.

Recipe 40:

Pasta with Tomato and Kale Stew

Serves: 3-4

Ingredients:

- 1 package 16 oz spaghetti, whole-grain and cooked
- 1 can tomatoes, diced

- 1 can corn, rinsed and drained
- 1 red onion, chopped
- 1 clove garlic, minced
- 1 bell pepper, seeded and chopped
- 1 jalapeno pepper, seeded and chopped
- ½ cup roasted cashews
- a bunch of kale
- pasta sauce

Preparation

Take a large skillet and sauté the onions and garlic on medium heat until lightly brown. Add the corn and continue to cook for 5 minutes then mix in bell peppers, jalapeno pepper and kale and cook for another 3 minutes. Add the tomatoes and sauce. Boil the spaghetti and serve with the stew on top. Spread the cashews on the stew.

Recipe 41:

Roasted Tomato and Eggplant Soup

Serves: 6

Ingredients:

- 1 large or 1 ½ pounds eggplant, chopped in chunks
- 3 pounds or 12 tomatoes, cored and sliced in halves
- ½ pound carrots, halved
- 1 can chickpeas 15oz, rinsed and drained
- 4 cups vegetable broth
- 1 onion, halved
- 10 garlic cloves, peeled
- 4 Tablespoons olive oil
- ½ cup fresh cilantro, chopped
- 2 teaspoons curry powder
- pepper and salt to taste

Preheat the oven at 425 degrees F.

Preparation

You need a rimmed baking sheet to roast different types at the same time.

Place the tomatoes, garlic, carrots, 2 Tablespoons olive oil, pepper and salt on a baking sheet and toss them together. Place the tomatoes with the cut sides facing downwards. All the ingredients should be spread in one layer. Place the chickpeas, eggplants,

2 Tablespoons oil, curry powder, pepper and salt on another baking sheet and toss them together. Spread them and then put both baking sheets in the oven. Roast for 45 minutes by which time they should be soft and tender. Turn the contents halfway after 22 ½ minutes so they can roast on both sides.

Remove from the oven and let everything cool slightly. Peel the tomatoes and puree them in a food processor or blender including all the juices.

Put the tomato puree in a pot, add the eggplant mixture and 3 cups vegetable broth or water then stir. Bring to a boil, cover and simmer over medium heat. Add 1 cup water if you need it lighter. Stir in pepper and salt to taste. Remove from heat. Serve with the fresh cilantro on top. You can eat the soup with bread, brown rice, pasta or noodles.

Recipe 42:

Toasted Eggplant (Aubergine) Ingredients:

- 3 eggplants, sliced without the stem

- 4 Tablespoons olive oil preferably extra-virgin olive oil
- ¼ cup chopped parsley
- 4 cloves of garlic, minced
- pinch of freshly ground pepper and salt

Preheat the oven at 400 degrees F.

Oil the baking sheet and arrange the sliced eggplants on it ensuring that they are on one layer. Apply more oil on the eggplants and sprinkle the garlic, pepper and salt. Bake for 25 minutes or less time when you notice that the eggplants have turned golden brown and tender. Remove the eggplants from the oven and let them cool. Serve with parsley sprinkled on top.

Preparation

Recipe 43:

Roasted French Beans

It is interesting how some vegetables become tasty when they are roasted. French beans can be roasted to add flavor.

Serves: 4-6

Ready in: 25 minutes

Ingredients:

- 2 pounds French beans
- 2 Tablespoons olive oil
- freshly ground pepper and salt to taste

Preheat the oven at 400 degrees F.

Trim the French beans after washing them thoroughly. Allow the water to drain from the beans and when they are dry spread them on a tray with your hands and toss them with olive oil. Sprinkle freshly ground pepper and salt on them. Bake for 25 minutes or less. Turn them on the other side after 15 or so minutes to roast the other side. Remove and serve them hot or if you like, at room temperature.

6: Smoothie Recipes

Smoothies are super-healthy drinks that contain antioxidants. They are loaded with carotenoids and flavonoids from a wide-spectrum of nature's best plant power recipes. These nutritious smoothies can be taken as delicious snacks or lunch. They are a combination of natural healthy and flavorful fruits, proteins, veggies and healthy fats. The fiber content in many fruits and vegetables make the consistency of some smoothies thick. You can add some water or add more of the juicy ingredient to make a drink you will enjoy. If the drink is too thin to your liking, add one peeled banana to the recipe.

Recipe 44:

Mango and Coconut Water Smoothie

Serving: 2

Ingredients:

- 2 cups peeled mango chunks
- 2 cups coconut water (unsweetened)
- 3 tablespoons freshly squeezed lime juice
- a pinch of cayenne powder

Preparation

Put the mango chunks into the blender; add coconut water, lime juice and a pinch of cayenne powder. Puree the mixture until it is smooth. Pour and serve in 2 glasses.

Nutrition value per serving: 159 calories, 39 g carbs, 3 g protein, 6 g fiber, 256 mg sodium, 1 g saturated fat, 0 unsaturated fats, 0 cholesterol.

Recipe 45:

Green Smoothie

Serving: 2

Ingredients:

- 1 apple, chopped
- 1 ripe banana
- 1 cup chopped collard greens without the stem
- 2 ½ cup water
- 1 cup parsley leaves

Preparation

Put all the ingredients into the blender including the water. Blend until the mixture is smooth. If you like a thinner smoothie, add some water.

Nutritional value per serving: 105 calories, 26 g carbs, 2 g protein, 4 g fiber, 32 mg sodium, 0 saturated fat, 0 unsaturated fat, 0 cholesterol.

Recipe 46:

Spinach and Pear Smoothie

Serves: 1 large serving or 2 medium servings

Ingredients:

- 1 cup almond milk
- ½ piece of ripe yellow pear
- ½ piece apple
- 1 cup baby spinach
- 1 frozen banana
- Ice cubes if you prefer it cold

Preparation

Pour all the ingredients in a blender and blend them together at high speed. Blend until smooth. Pour in a large glass or in 2 medium glasses and serve.

Recipe 47:

Mango, Orange and Carrot Herbal Smoothie

Serving: 2

Ingredients:

- 1 cup peeled mango chunks, frozen
- 1 cup fresh orange juice, squeezed
- 1 cup fresh carrot juice
- ¼ cup mixture of fresh herbs like basil, mint and others.

Preparation

Put all the ingredients into the blender including the fresh herbs. Blend until the mixture is smooth.

Nutritional value per serving: 225 calories, 56 g carbs, 3 g protein, 5 g fiber, 35 mg sodium, 0 saturated fat, 0 unsaturated fat, 0 cholesterol.

Recipe 48:

Orange and Pumpkin Spice Smoothie

Ingredients:

- 3 tablespoons cooked or canned pumpkin
- ½ cup soy or almond milk

- ½ tablespoon pumpkin spice
- ¼ cup orange juice
- 1 peeled orange
- Sliced cucumber and lemon pieces

Preparation

Mix all the ingredients in a blender and process until the mixture is smooth. Serve in 2 glasses.

Recipe 49:

Kiwi Smoothie

Serving: 2

Ingredients:

- 4 ripe kiwi chunks, peeled
- ½ cup fresh orange juice, squeezed
- 1 cup ice
- 1 tablespoon of agave nectar

Preparation

Halve the kiwi fruits and put all the ingredients into the blender including the ice. Blend until the mixture is smooth.

Nutritional value per serving: 142 calories, 35 g carbs, 2 g protein, 4 g fiber, 5 mg sodium, 0 saturated fat, 0 unsaturated fat, 0 cholesterol.

Recipe 50:

Carrot, Apple, Orange and Ginger Smoothie

Serving: 2

Ingredients:

- 1 cup fresh carrot juice
- 1 peeled apple without core, chopped
- 1 cup fresh orange juice, squeezed
- 1 teaspoon fresh ginger, grated

Preparation

Put all the ingredients into the blender. Blend until the mixture is smooth.

Nutritional value per serving: 174 calories, 41 g carbs, 2 g protein, 3 g fiber, 37 mg sodium, 0 saturated fat, 0 unsaturated fat, 0 cholesterol.

Recipe 51:

Blueberry and Almond (Butter) Smoothie

Serving: 2

Ingredients:

- 1 ½ cups of blueberries or strawberries or blueberries, frozen
- 1 ripe banana
- 3 cups of water
- 3 tablespoons of almond butter
- 3 pitted dates
- 2 tablespoons of flaxseed
- 1 tablespoon of freshly squeezed lemon juice

Preparation

Put all the ingredients into the blender including the water. Blend until the mixture is smooth. If you like a thinner smoothie, add some more water little by little.

Nutritional value per serving: 405 calories, 63 g carbs, 7 g protein, 10 g fiber, 117 mg sodium, 2 g saturated fat, 15 g unsaturated fat, 0 cholesterol.

Recipe 52:

Pomegranate and Berry Smoothie

Serving: 2

Ingredients:

- 1 cup pomegranate juice, unsweetened
- 1 cup mixed berries, frozen (9 oz)
- 1 cup water

Preparation

Mix pomegranate juice, water and the mixed berries into the blender. Blend until the mixture is smooth.

Nutritional value per serving: 130 calories, 34 g carbs, 1.5 g protein, 4 g fiber, 19 mg sodium, 1 g saturated fat, 0 unsaturated fat, 0 cholesterol.

Recipe 53:

Carrot and Beet Smoothie

Carrots are rich in Vitamin A antioxidants and carotenoids.

Serving: 2

Ingredients:

- ½ cup carrots, peeled and chopped
- 1 apple, chopped
- ½ cup red beets, peeled and chopped

- 1 ripe pear, chopped
- 1 tablespoon fresh lemon or lime juice, squeezed
- 1 teaspoon fresh ginger, minced
- 2 cups water

Preparation

Combine all the ingredients in the blender including the water. Blend until the mixture is smooth. Alternatively, steam the carrots and beet for 10 minutes and let them cool before you combine the ingredients in the blender.

Nutritional value per serving: 135 calories, 35 g carbs, 2 g protein, 7 g fiber, 62 mg sodium, 0 saturated fat, 0 unsaturated fat, 0 cholesterol.

Recipe 54:

Orange, Raspberry and Blueberry Smoothie

Serving: 2

Ingredients:

- 2 orange chunks, peeled and seeds removed
- 1 cup raspberries, frozen
- 1 cup blueberries, frozen

Preparation

Combine all the ingredients in the blender. Blend until the mixture is smooth.

Nutritional value per serving: 132 calories, 34 g carbs, 2 g protein, 3 g fiber, 2 mg sodium, 0 saturated fat, 0 unsaturated fat, 0 cholesterol.

Recipe 55:

Chilly Strawberry Smoothie

Serves: 2

Ready in: 6 minutes

Ingredients:

- 10 medium strawberries, hulled
- 1 cup non-dairy milk
- 2 Tablespoons maple syrup or vegan sugar
- 1 teaspoon vanilla extract
- 6 crushed ice cubes

Preparation Put 8 strawberries, non-dairy milk, maple syrup, vanilla extract and the ice in a blender. Blend until smooth. Serve in 2 glasses and garnish with the remaining 2 strawberries.

Recipe 56:

Delicious Strawberry and Banana Smoothie

- 10 oz fresh or frozen strawberries, stemmed
- 2 ripe bananas, peeled and sliced
- 3 tablespoons agape syrup or vegan sugar
- ¾ cup soy milk or almond milk or coconut water

Optional

- ice cubes
- vanilla or almond extract

Place all the washed ingredients in a blender and process until smooth. Serve and garnish with whole strawberries.

Recipe 57:

Strawberry and Orange Smoothie

- 1cup fresh or frozen strawberries or raspberries, stemmed
- 1 cup orange juice
- ¾ cup soy milk or almond milk or coconut water

Place all the washed ingredients in a blender and process until smooth. Serve and garnish with whole strawberries or raspberries.

Recipe 58:

Orange and Pumpkin Spice Smoothie

Serving: 4

Ingredients:

- 3 tablespoons cooked or canned pumpkin
- ½ cup soy or almond milk
- ½ tablespoon pumpkin spice
- ¼ cup orange juice
- 1 peeled orange
- Sliced cucumber and lemon pieces

Preparation

Mix all the ingredients in a blender and process until the mixture is smooth. Serve in 2 glasses.

Recipe 59:

Soy and Strawberry Smoothie

Serving: 2

Ingredients:

- 1 cup of soy milk
- 2 cups strawberries, frozen (8 oz)
- 1 ripe banana
- 2 tablespoons of honey

Preparation:

Combine all the ingredients in the blender including the water. Blend until the mixture is smooth.

Nutritional value per serving: 235 calories, 52 g carbs, 5 g protein, 5 g fiber, 67 mg sodium, 0 saturated fat, 2 g unsaturated fat, 0 cholesterol.

Recipe 60:

Banana and Ginger Smoothie

Serving: 2

Ingredients:

- 1 cup of fresh orange juice
- 1 teaspoon fresh ginger, grated
- 1 ripe banana
- 1 cup ice
- 2 tablespoons of honey

Preparation

Combine all the ingredients in the blender including the water. Blend until the mixture is smooth.

Nutritional value per serving: 174 calories, 44 g carbs, 2 g protein, 2 g fiber, 3 mg sodium, 0 saturated fat, 0 unsaturated fat, 0 cholesterol.

7: Juices Recipes

The following are nutrient-rich juice recipes which are easy to make. You can add watermelon or other watery fruits or a little water to any of the juices if you need the consistency to be thinner. You don't have to buy a juicer if you don't have one, use your blender. Most juices have natural beautiful tastes that you and your kids will love.

Fruit and vegetable juices help to cleanse, energize, build and regenerate our bodies. When you take a combination of fresh fruits and vegetable live juices you get all the vitamins, minerals, enzymes, proteins and healthy fats that vitalize your body. These juices and smoothies have a rejuvenating effect on your health helping you to get prevention and healing of many illnesses and diseases.

Many of the fruits and vegetables used in these juices are packed with phytonutrients, antioxidants, chlorophyll, beta carotene, essential fatty acids, iron, Vitamin A, B vitamins, Vitamin C, Vitamin K, and Vitamin E among other health benefits especially if they are consumed raw.

Recipe 61:

Kiwi, Grapefruit and Orange Juice

You can boost your immunity with these fruits which are so rich in Vitamin C and other antioxidants. Citrus fruits awaken you up and vitalize you in the morning and within no time you will find yourself out of the door.

Serves: 2

Ingredients

- 3 kiwis 12 0z
- 2 oranges 10 oz
- 1 grapefruit 14 oz

Peel all the kiwis, grapefruit and orange fruits and cut them in chunks. Put the chunks in a juicer or blender and puree until smooth. Strain the juice and serve. The juice can be kept in the fridge for 2 days. The contents may settle at the bottom, so, shake before you serve.

Recipe 62:

Fresh Pomegranate and Apple Juice

Ingredients:

- 1 pomegranate without the seeds
- 1 apple, cored

This is a great punch for anyone searching for an anti-oxidant juice. Pomegranates are a favorite in many household and kids like them too. You can imagine how awesome the juice of pomegranates and apples would taste. Drinking squeezed pomegranates when they are fresh gives, you that refreshing feeling.

Recipe 63:

Strawberry, Orange and Grapes Juice

Ingredients:

- 1 cup strawberries
- 1 orange, peeled and seeded
- 1 cup red grapes

Recipe 64:

Watermelon and Apple Juice

Ingredients:

- 3 slices of watermelon, peeled
- 1 apple, cored

Many juice lovers look forward to summer when most fruits especially watermelon are in season so they can extract juice. Try and juice even watermelon alone and you will feel refreshed.

Peel the watermelon and cut into medium-sized chunks. The watermelon seeds aid in digestion, so blend them together. Remove the core of the apple and cut it also. Put the ingredients in a fruit juice extractor or blender and blend until smooth. Serve.

Recipe 65:

Carrot and Grape Juice/Desert

Ingredients:

- 2 carrots, peeled and sliced
- ½ cup green grapes
- 2 peaches, pitted
- 2 apricots, pitted

Start by pitting both the apricots and peaches. Put them n a blender. Peel and slice the carrots and add them to the blender. Add the grapes and blend until smooth. You may serve this as a desert since the consistency is thick.

Recipe 66:

Apple and Strawberry Juice

Ingredients:

- 2 medium apples
- 1 cup strawberries
- ½ lemon, juiced

Recipe 67:

Cucumber, Cilantro and Kale Green Juice

Serves: 2

Ingredients:

- 1 large cucumber
- 1 medium apple, cored
- 1 medium stalk of celery
- 6 big leaves of kale
- 2 handfuls of cilantro
- 1 lime, peeled

Cut the kale and celery and put in a juice extractor. Cut the cucumber, apples and cilantro and add to the juicer. Cut the peeled lime into quarter without the core. Juice all the ingredients together. Sieve and serve in 2 glasses.

Recipe 68:

Berry and Mango Drink

Serves: 2Ingredients:

- 1 cup fresh strawberries, halved or frozen and thawed
- 1 cup fresh blueberries, or frozen and thawed
- 2 mangos, peeled and chopped
- ¼ cup of water

Put the strawberries, blueberries, mango and the water in a blender and blend until smooth. Strain and serve in 2 glasses or keep in the fringe up to 2 days. Always shake before serving. Garnish with pieces of mango, strawberries or blueberries.

Recipe 69:

Green Juice Cleanser

Health vitality organic

Serves: 2

Ready by: 10 minutes or less

Ingredients:

- 1 large cucumber
- 1 medium apple, cored
- 1 medium stalk of celery
- 6 big leaves of kale
- 2 handfuls of cilantro
- 1 lime, peeled

Cut the kale, cilantro and celery and put in a juice extractor. Cut the cucumber and apples and add to the juicer. Cut the peeled lemon into quarters without the seeds or 1 tablespoon of lime juice and put in the juicer or blender. Juice all the ingredients together. Sieve and serve in 2 glasses.

Recipe 70:

Green Power Plant Juice

Serves: 3-4

Ready by: 10 minutes or less

Ingredients:

- 2 medium cucumbers, sliced

- 2 medium apples, cored
- 2 cups spinach, chopped
- ½ inch ginger root, freshly ground
- 1 medium stalk of celery, chopped
- ½ cup parsley, chopped
- ½ lemon, juice
- 1 lime, juice
- crushed ice cubes or water

Optional

- Carrot
- banana

Put all the ingredients in a juice extractor or blender. Blend until it is smooth. If you are using a juice extractor, sieve and serve. Add some water or unsweetened fresh juice if the juice is too thick to make the consistency you are happy with.

Recipe 71:

Tropical Delight Juice

Ingredients:

- 2 mangoes, peeled
- 1pinneaple, peeled and cored

- 1 cup strawberry

Peel the rind of the pineapple and remove the core. Peel the mango also. After peeling the fruits, cut them in chunks. Put them in a juicer or blender and juice all the ingredients together. Serve.

Recipe 72:

Refresher Juice

Ingredients:

- 2 leaves of kale
- 1 pear, peeled
- 2 apples, cored
- ½ lemon, peeled and seeded
- ½ inch ginger, grated
- a handful of cilantro
- a handful of spinach

Remove the hard stem of the kale and spinach. Cut with your hands and put in the blender. Add the other ingredients and blend until smooth then serve.

Recipe 73:

Apple, Plum and Pear Juice

Ingredients:

- 2 apples, cored
- 2 plums, pitted
- 2 pears, cored

Put all the ingredients in a juicer or blender and blend until smooth. Serve.

Recipe 74:

Natural Berry Juice

Berries have anti-aging antioxidants

Ingredients:

- 1 apple, cored
- 2 cups strawberries
- 2 cups raspberries or less
- 2 cups blueberries

Remove the core of the apple and chop it. Put in a juicer or blender and add the berries. Blend until smooth.

Recipe 75:

Apple, Berry, Mango and Orange Juice

Ingredients:

- 1 apple, cored
- 2 cups strawberries
- 1 cup raspberries
- 2 cups blueberries
- 1 mango, peeled
- 1 orange, peeled without the seeds

Core the apple and cut it, the mango and orange in chunks. Put in the juicer and add the berries. Process until it is smooth.

Recipe 76:

Apple, Carrot and Tangerine Juice

Ingredients:

- 2 tangerines, peeled
- 2 carrots, sliced
- 1 tablespoon of flaxseed
- 1 apple, cored
- ¼ inch piece of ginger, minced

Put all the ingredients in a juice extractor or blender. Blend until it is smooth. If you are using a juice extractor, sieve and serve. Add some water or unsweetened fresh juice if the juice is too thick to make the consistency you are happy with.

You can substitute chai seeds for flaxseed if you like. The juice will still be awesome.

Recipe 77:

Cucumber and Apple Juice

Ingredients:

- ½ cucumbers, sliced
- 5 apples, cored

When you juice cucumbers and apples together, the juice is so refreshing. They say that "An apple a day keeps the doctors away" You may find the taste of cucumber to be strong although it is cooling, so, put only half of it. Cucumber is a cleanser and it aids elimination of toxins from the system. If you want to detoxify, add more cucumbers.

Recipe 78:

Cranberries, Apple and Carrot Juice

Ingredients:

- 2 apples, cored
- 2 carrots, sliced
- ¾ cup cranberries

Cranberries are a great nutrient for the liver and bladder.

Recipe 79:

Carrot, Orange and Melon Juice

Ingredients:

- 2 oranges
- 1 carrot
- Half a melon

Peel the carrot and cut it in slices. Remove the rind of the orange and cut it into chunks. Peel the melon and slice it also. Juice all the ingredients together.

Recipe 80:

Orange, Strawberry and Grapes Juice

Ingredients:

- 1 orange, peeled
- 2 apples, cored
- 2 carrots, sliced
- 1 cup red grapes
- 1 cup strawberries

Remove the rind of the orange and cut it in chunks. Juice the orange, apples, grapes and strawberries together. Strain and serve

Recipe 81:

Apple, Carrot, Citrus and Greens Juice

Ingredients:

- 2 green apples, cored
- 2 carrots, sliced
- 1 bunch celery
- 3 kale leaves
- 1 big handful of parsley leaves
- 1 lemon
- 1 lime
- small fresh ginger

Place all the ingredients in a juicer and process until smooth. Serve in glasses and enjoy.

Recipe 82:

Fresh Watermelon Juice

Watermelon juice quenches thirst especially in those summer days. Watermelon is 90% water

Serves: 5

Ingredients:

- 2 kg peeled watermelon, seeded
- 2 Tablespoons fresh lemon juice
- 1 Tablespoon ginger, grated thinly
- ice cubes

Preparation

Cut the seeded watermelon in chunks and put them in a blender. Add the lemon juice and ginger and blend until smooth. Sieve into a jug and serve with ice.

Recipe 83:

Carrot, Tomato and Orange Juice with Garlic

Ingredients:

- 1 pound cherry tomatoes
- 2 teaspoons garlic, minced
- 1 orange
- 2 carrots

Put all the ingredients in a juice extractor or blender. Blend until it is smooth. If you are using a juice extractor, sieve and serve. Add some water or unsweetened fresh juice if the juice is too thick to make the consistency you are happy with.

Recipe 84:

Strawberry, Apple, Cucumber and Carrot Juice

Ingredients:

- 6 fresh strawberries, hulled
- 2 medium carrots, peeled and sliced
- 1 cucumber sliced
- 1 red apple, cored and chopped

Optional

- ice cubes

Process the strawberries, carrots, cucumber and apple in a juicer or blender, until smooth. Put ice cubes in 2 glasses and pour the juice. Serve the refreshing, healthy drink immediately.

Nutritional value per serving: 69 calories, 15 g carbs, 1 g protein, 1 g fiber, 30 mg sodium, 0 saturated fat, 0 unsaturated fat, 0 cholesterol, 249 mg potassium.

Recipe 85:

Apple, Kale, Celery and Citrus Juice

Ingredients:

- 6 kale leaves, stemmed
- 4 celery stalks
- 2 apples
- 1 cucumber
- ½ lemon
- ½ inch fresh ginger, ground

This juice is a good cleanser. It cleanses the system and provides nutrients to the body.

Before you put any raw fruits and vegetables in the juicer or blender, wash them thoroughly. Blend the ingredients or process them until they are smooth. Use a platter to remove any contents holding on the sides of the juicer and push them in the middle. Some may settle in the bottom so you should shake thoroughly before serving. There are some people who prefer to sieve their juices while others enjoy thin consistency. Do whatever pleases you and enjoy. Some juices and smoothies are great when they are served chilly with ice while others are enjoyed when they are at room temperature.

You can change any ingredients to suit your taste. Some people like juicing everything without peeling the rinds or peels and with the seeds on in order to get wholesome foods. Everyone is different and what works for one person may not work for the other.

Take smoothies and juices every day if you need to stay healthy. Make different green juices for cleansing your system, fruit juices to add the nutrients the body requires and a mixture of plant power foods as your nutritional powerhouse. Citrus fruits like oranges, grapefruits, lemons and limes are full of Vitamin C and they are great cleansers.

8: Salads

Recipe 86:

Chicken Pea, Tomato and Feta Salad

Serves: 2

Time: 10 minutes

Ingredients:

- ½ cup canned chickpeas, drained
- 1 cup ripe tomatoes, quartered
- 2 tablespoon fresh lemon juice, squeezed
- ½ cup feta, crumbled
- 1 tablespoon oregano
- 2 tablespoons olive oil
- Salt and pepper to taste

Preparation

Combine the chickpeas, tomatoes, feta, lemon juice and olive oil in a bowl and mix. Add oregano and lemon juice. Season the salad with salt and pepper to give it taste.

Recipe 87:

Cauliflower Salad (Warm)

This delicious cauliflower salad is served warm. You can substitute roasted almonds with cashews or any other nuts that you prefer to make your salad a delicacy.

Serves: 4

Time: 50 minutes

Ingredients:

- 1 medium cauliflower, florets
- 50 g of baby spinach
- 1 red onion, sliced
- a small bunch of dill
- 3 tablespoons of toasted almonds or cashews, flaked
- 3 tablespoons of sherry vinegar
- 3 tablespoons of raisins
- 2 tablespoons of olive oil
- 1 ½ tablespoons maple syrup
- salt to taste

Preparation

Roast the cauliflower sparkled with the olive oil for 15 minutes. Add the onions and stir then keep roasting until the cauliflower becomes tender. Stir in the raisins, vinegar, salt and maple syrup.

You can serve the cauliflower crunchy or soft which depends on your preference. Remove from the oven when ready and combine with spinach, almond and dressing. Serve the salad warm.

Recipe 88:

Sweet Potato Spicy Salad

Serves: 6-8

Ingredients:

- 1 pound sweet colored potatoes, peeled and cubed
- 4 trimmed stallions, sliced
- 1 red onion, sliced
- 3 cups cooked corn, fresh or frozen
- ½ jalapeno pepper, sliced
- 2 tablespoons vegetable oil
- 1 tablespoon cumin

- ½ tablespoon cayenne pepper
- Salt and pepper to taste

Garnish

- ¼ cup cilantro, chopped

Dressing

- 1 clove of garlic, minced
- ¼ cup vegetable oil
- 1 fresh lime, juice
- salt and pepper

Preparation

Start by pre-heating the oven to 400 degrees F. Take a baking sheet lined with aluminum foil and lay the sweet potatoes sprinkled with salt and pepper, vegetable oil, cayenne pepper and cumin. Turn the sweet potatoes once when they are baked on one side. The baking should take about 25 minutes. Keep them aside once they are ready for them to cool.

Toss the stallions, cooked corn, jalapeno and bell peppers and combine them.

Whisk the dressing ingredients together in a bowl to make a citrus dressing. Combine the potatoes with the dressing and then garnish with cilantro.

Recipe 89:

Apple, Celery and Walnut Salad

Serves: 4

Ingredients:

- 4 apples, cored and thinly sliced
- 2 sticks of celery, thinly sliced
- 1 red onion, thinly sliced
- 1/3 cup of apple cider vinegar
- ½ teaspoon fennel seeds, ground
- ½ cup walnuts, sliced

Preparation

Put the fennel seeds and apple cider vinegar in a bowl and mix thoroughly. Combine apples, celery, walnuts and onions in a bowl. Add the fennel seeds and vinegar dressing. Mix gently and serve.

Recipe 90:

Carrot, Peach, Apricot and Grape Desert

Ingredients:

- 2 carrots, peeled and sliced
- 2 peaches, pitted
- 2 apricots, pitted
- ½ cup green grapes

Preparation

Start by pitting the apricots and peaches and cutting them in mouthful sizes. Peel and slice the carrots in small sized. Garnish with the grapes. You may also blend the ingredients to serve as a desert since the consistency is thick.

Recipe 91:

Cucumbers, Tomatoes Salad with Dill Dressing

Serves: 6

Ready in: 30 Minutes

Ingredients:

- 2 medium cucumbers, sliced
- 2 red tomatoes, sliced
- ½ cup red onions, sliced
- 2 Tablespoon vegetable oil

- ¼ cup balsamic vinegar or cider vinegar
- ½ teaspoon fresh dill, chopped (or 1 teaspoon dried dill)
- ¼ teaspoon black pepper, ground
- 1 teaspoon sugar
- ½ teaspoon salt

Preparation

Take a bowl and make the dressing by mixing sugar, salt, vegetable oil, dill, vinegar and pepper. You can use dried dill but you will need the double the quantity used. Add the crunchy cucumbers, tomatoes and onions and mix all the ingredients together. Let the salad stand for 15 minutes before serving so the flavors can mix together. Serve with your favorite dish.

Recipe 92:

Cucumber, Cilantro and Kale Green Salad

Serves: 2

Ingredients:

- 1 large cucumber, sliced
- 1 medium apple, cored

- 1 medium stalk of celery, trimmed
- 3 big leaves of kale, stem removed and thinly cut
- 2 handfuls of cilantro, chopped
- 1 handful of baby spinach, chopped

Preparation

You can use scissors to cut the hard stems of the kale leaves then cut them thinly with a knife. Add baby spinach to make the kale soft. Cut the celery and cilantro. Slice the cucumber in rounds and the apples in lengthwise wedges. Mix all the ingredients and serve.

Recipe 93:

Green Power Plant Salad

Serves: 3-4

Ready by: 10 minutes

Ingredients:

- 2 medium cucumbers, sliced
- 2 medium apples, cored
- 2 cups baby spinach, chopped
- 2 carrot, sliced

- 1 medium stalk of celery, chopped
- ½ cup parsley, chopped
- ½ squeezed fresh lemon juice
- 1 squeezed fresh lime juice

Preparation

Slice the cucumbers, carrots and apples. Chop the spinach, celery and parsley. Mix all the ingredients in a bowl. You can squeeze the juice of both the lemon and lime and mix with the salad to add Vitamin C from the citrus.

Recipe 94:

Grilled Vegetable Salad

You can have your vegetables grilled to add flavor to them.

Serves: 6

Ready in: 30 minutes

Ingredients:

- 2 zucchini, trimmed and halved lengthwise
- 2 yellow squash, trimmed and halved lengthwise
- 1 pound asparagus, trimmed on the ends

- 1 red onion, sliced
- 2 red bell peppers, seeded and halved
- 1 teaspoon mustard
- 1 clove garlic, minced
- ½ cup extra virgin olive oil
- pepper and salt to taste

Preparation

Pre-heat the grill in medium heat and arrange the zucchini, squash, asparagus, onions and bell pepper on a grill tray. Grill the vegetables until they become tender which should take about 15 minutes but if you like them a bit crunch 10 minutes should be enough.

Prepare the dressing with mustard, garlic, extra virgin oil, pepper and salt. You can add some wine vinegar if you like.

Remove the vegetables from the grill once they are ready and cut them ready for serving. Serve with the dressing either warm or at room temperature whichever you prefer.

Recipe 95:

Crunchy Cauliflower Salad

Serves: 4

Ingredients:

- 1 medium cauliflower, in florets
- 50 g of baby spinach, chopped
- 1 red onions, sliced
- 3 tablespoons raisins
- 3 tablespoons almonds, roasted
- 1-2 tablespoons maple syrup
- 1 tablespoon olive oil

Preparation

Steam the cauliflower in medium heat in a skillet until they are crunchy. Remove from the heat and keep aside to cool a little. Add the chopped baby spinach and all the other ingredients and toss to make a crunchy salad. Serve it warm or at room temperature.

Recipe 96:

Refresher Salad

Ingredients:

- 1 pear, peeled and chopped
- 2 apples, cored and chopped

- 2 leaves of kale, without the hard stem
- ½ lemon, seeded
- 1/4 inch ginger, minced
- a handful of fresh cilantro
- a handful of baby spinach

Preparation

Remove the hard stem of the kale with scissors and cut it thinly. Peel and chop the pear, core and chop the apple then cut cilantro and spinach. Add the ginger and mix all the ingredients. You can squeeze the lemon juice to add taste to the salad.

Recipe 97:

Cucumber and Apple Juice

Ingredients:

- ½ cucumbers, sliced
- 5 apples, cored

Preparation

When you juice cucumbers and apples together, the juice is so refreshing. They say that "An apple a day keeps the doctors away" You may find the taste of cucumber to be strong although it is cooling, so, put only half of it. Cucumber is a cleanser and it aids elimination of toxins from the system. If you want to detoxify, add more cucumbers.

9: Jam and Sauce Recipes

Recipe 98:

Pear and Pomegranate Jam

Serving: 1 jar

Ingredients:

- 2 cups pear, chopped
- 2 fresh pomegranate juice, strained
- ¼ cup of pomegranate seeds
- ¼ cup of rose wine
- 2 cups of sugar or less
- a bit of lemon rind, grated
- pinch of rosemary or lavender, minced
- 1 teaspoon of fruit pectin
- ½ teaspoon of plant based butter

Preparation

Mix the chopped pear, pomegranate, sugar, and rose wine together in a saucepan and put the mixture on medium heat. Let it boil and keep stirring the sugar until it dissolves. Simmer for 25-30 minutes or until the pear becomes tender.

Remove from the heat and use a potato masher to mash the mixture.

Recipe 99:

Walnut Sauce

- 1/2 cup walnuts, finely chopped
- 1 ½ cups vegan milk i.e. soy milk
- 1 fresh bay leaves
- 2 tablespoons olive oil, organic
- 1 teaspoon vegan sugar
- 1 ½ Tbs. whole wheat flour
- pepper and salt

Garnish

- fresh parsley

Preparation

Put soy milk, walnuts, garlic and by leaves on a saucepan and cook, stirring regularly. Remove from the heat when it is about to boil.

Take another saucepan and put the oil, add the sugar and wheat flour and cook for 3 minutes on low heat. Pour the above mixture without the bay leaves and mix thoroughly. Cover and simmer for 25 minutes. Season the sauce with pepper and salt. Remove from heat. Serve and garnish with parsley.

Add the pomegranate seeds and plant based butter of your choice to the mixture and boil. Add fruit pectin and boil again while you stir consistently. Remove the jam from the heat and add rosemary and lemon rind. Stir and let it cool to the room temperature. Pour in a glass jar, cover with lid and keep in the fridge overnight. Serve on bread. The taste is delicious.

Recipe 100:

Cranberry Sauce

- 2 packages of organically-grown cranberries, fresh
- 8 dates, pitted
- 1orange, peeled and chopped
- 1lemon, peeled and chopped
- pinch of cinnamon
- 1 cup water
- 2 Tbs. maple syrup (optional)

Soak the dates for 1 hour in filtered water put cranberries on a saucepan with water and cook over medium heat until the cranberries are tender and soft. Add pitted dates and the citrus fruits, cinnamon and maple syrup then cook for additional 5 minutes. Mix all the ingredients in a blender and puree.

Conclusion

You now understand what plant based diet can do for your health and what a positive influence it can have in our daily lives. Plant Power Foods are rich in nutrients that the body needs to function properly. It fights off diseases from attacking the immune system.

Nature has all that we require to live healthy lives boosting with vibrant energy. Contrary to popular belief, plant based recipes can be delicious than what most people expect because they have natural flavors that are hard to find in processed foods loaded with refined sugars and other ingredients to make them tasty.

The secret with Plant Power Foods is that they add nutrients to the body without overloading our systems with toxins.

Thank you for downloading this book. I hope you enjoy it!

10074654R00070

Printed in Great Britain
by Amazon.co.uk, Ltd.,
Marston Gate.